Sex Positions Handbook

A Guide To 25 Exotic Sex Positions
That Gives Multiple Orgasms

LAURA WHITE

ISBN-13: 978-1530037018

ISBN-10: 1530037018

DEDICATION

To all who desire to live life to the fullest!

TABLE OF CONTENT

INTRODUCTION

Sex and making love can be a herculean task, if you don't know how to go about it. This is a book founded by a great passion to see lovers enjoy quality sex in a creative way and it has been written in simple words that can be easily understood by anyone.

Many lovers are limited to two sex positions or more in their sex lives, and some other lovers are fast becoming bored with how boring those few sex positions are turning out to be, and how boring their sex life might be turning out.

This book was written for you, to spice up your sex life. It contains exotic sex position that you should take time out to try out. Enjoy as you read through this book and have fun with your lover. Happy reading.

Carnal Crisscross

The woman starts by lying on her side with her arms above her head. The man on his side and his body perpendicular to the woman's, the woman slowly raises her top leg and let him inch his lower body between her legs. Once the couple is joined at the groin, the man should grab her shoulders while she anchors herself on the floor. The couple will need to hold on tight for this stellar trip!

Cross Sex Position

This position is different from the Scissors positions because the man lies at right angles to the woman. With the lower body of the man under both the woman's bent legs; the woman being laid back in the Missionary position. This angle decreases chances of skin contact but allows more unique penetration angle

Deck Chair Sex Position

In this position, the woman lays on her back, and pivots her hips so that her legs is in the air, and then she bends her knees while the man enters from a kneeling position while supporting some of his weight on the woman's legs. This position is a favorite of many men because of the sense of power that comes from folding their lover; this position doesn't leave the receiver out of the fun. When the man leans on the woman's legs, it better improves the angle of penetration to better target the g-spot, and increase satisfaction of the woman

Deep Impact Sex Position

This sex position is a variation of the Deep Stick sex position, but it is easier as the man kneels by the side of the bed or couch thereby lining up more easily with the woman. To get into position, the woman lies on her back with her legs resting on the shoulders of the man, who penetrates his woman from a kneeling position. This position also stays true to its name, meaning the man can thrust in with all intensity, unless of course he is too big. Any height difference or discomforts on the side of the man can be easily be fixed using pillows.

Downstroke Sex Positions

This position is also a variation of the Deep Stick sex position, but it is easier as the man crouches by the side of the bed, sofa or couch. So he lines up more easily with the woman. To get into this position, the woman will need to lie on her back with her legs resting on the shoulders of the man, the man then penetrates from a standing position. But due to the higher position of the man this variation is not as intimate as either the Deep Stick sex position or its other family the Deep Impact sex position.

Drill Sex Position

In this position, the woman lies on her back and wraps her legs around her man who mounts her from above.

Although it looks very similar to the Missionary position, the raised legs of the woman makes a significant improvement in the penetration angle as well as the intimacy, therefore making it a good first step for improving the sometimes monotonous starting position.

Exposed Eagle Sex Position

This position might just be one of the hardest positions to perform. It requires great flexibility and strength. If you don't have this gym or yoga expertise, then the couple is in for a pretty sore time!

The best way to get into this position is to start out in the Cowgirl position. This means that the woman needs to be on top of her man with her knees on either side of him. She then lies backwards until her back is resting on her man's thighs and knees while she is still on her knees. He can raise his knees if she isn't flexible enough so she is more upright. The man now needs to raise his upper body so that he is in a seated position. He can then put his arms behind him to support himself or he can put them around the woman's back.

Hang Loose Sex Position

This position is really an easy one to perform. It is a variation of the regular Missionary position. You don't have to sleep in the gym or be a work out expert to get into this position

The couple starts off in the regular Missionary position, instead of them lying with their heads by where the pillows are and their feet near the end of the bed, the couple lies across the bed. Lying across the bed will give both of them far less space. To overcome this, the woman should position herself so that her head and part of her shoulders are hanging over the edge of the bed. Her man will also be hanging over the bed, so he will need to extend his arms outwards and put his hands on the ground to support himself.

This sex position got its name from the fact that the couples are literally hanging over the edge of your bed.

Italian Hanger Sex Position

This sex position is great for hitting the woman's G-Spot while, and she also has a cool 'exposed' and slightly submissive feeling to it. It is very easy to make a transition from the missionary position into the Italian Hanger. The woman just needs to lie on her back

As the man is having the regular missionary sex, he would then need to get to his knees and bring them quite close to the woman, which will force her legs apart. When he is on his knees, he then needs to put his hands under the woman's bum and hips and lift them up. To help him out with raising her bum and hips, the woman bends her knees and plant her feet on the bed. This will allow her to push her waist or hips into the air.

The launch Pad sex position

It is one great way to get into a synchronistic sexual flow, whether the couple opts for deep and powerful thrusts or gentle rocking. It's also helps if couples want to achieve deep penetration and the massage of the woman's G-spot.

As in Deep Stick sex position, the woman lies on her back and raises her hips; the man now kneels down in front. Once the man penetrates the woman and begins to thrust, the woman's hips rise and fall in beautiful rhythm to every thrust. A positional aid can be placed underneath the buttocks of the woman, to help her maintain the elevation of her hips.

The woman's leg positions can be modified in many ways, like: bringing both legs over to a side, the man raising them over his shoulders, or keeping her feet together and spreading her knees wide. The woman can also place her feet on the chest of her man to bear some of his weight so that her man can lean over top of her legs; this gives a difference in sensation.

Missionary 180 Sex Position

This Sex Position is like a combination of two sex positions, the regular Missionary and the Betty Rocker Sex positions. For the man it will require quite a bit of flexibility in his penis to be able perform the position.

The woman starts by lying down on her back with her legs fairly spread out. The man will then lie down on top of her. But instead of the couples lying facing each other, the man will be lying head-to-toe with his legs spread out, resting on either side of you on the bed. The man now slowly and carefully pushes his penis downwards so that he can thrust into the woman's vagina. This will definitely put a lot of strain on the suspensory ligaments in the man's penis, hence the need for a reasonable level of flexibility, so he needs to be extra careful while doing this.

Pirate's Bounty Sex Position

In this sex position, the woman lies on her back with one of her legs resting on the man's shoulder; the other leg is wrapped around the man's thigh (the ship mast). The man penetrates her vagina from a kneeling position. Fairly easier to perform than its near cousin the Deep Stick, this position holds true to its name, meaning that the man can penetrate with every ounce of strength he has, unless of course he is too big. Any genital altitude difference should be corrected easily, by the use of pillows.

The Playing Of the Cello Sex Position

This position is a really enjoyable one for the woman. The reason it has the name is because the man will look almost like he is playing the cello with the woman's legs.

The woman lies on her back and raises her legs so that the legs are pointing towards the ceiling. Her man is then positioned upright, on his knees and penetrates the woman while facing her. The woman now rests both of her legs on just one of his shoulders, either the right or the left shoulder. The man now wraps one arm around the woman's feet and lower leg, while wrapping his other arm around her thighs, which makes the man look like he's playing the cello with his woman's legs, hence the name playing the Cello sex position.

Right Angle Sex Position

It is a really easy to perform sex position and doesn't require so much flexibility.

The woman starts by lying down on her back and pointing her feet towards the ceiling. She doesn't have to worry so much about keeping her legs perfectly straight. The man then sits down on the bed with his legs spread open. He should be facing his woman and sitting down on the bed just below her vagina with his legs in front of him on either side of the woman's body. The man now grabs her legs and lifts her up and towards him. He can then thrust into her.

The Right Angle got its name from the idea that the couple will be making a 90 degree angle, which is a right angle with your bodies in this sex position.

Sandwich Sex Position

This position is a little like the combination if two sex positions, the Viennese Oyster and Drill positions. It requires a little bit of flexibility and strength on the part of the woman.

The woman lies down on her back and let her man thrust into her as he would while in the Missionary position; on top. But instead of just resting her legs on the bed like she would in the missionary, she brings them towards herself while keeping them open. Her man's arms should usually be around her shoulders on the bed, but he would now have to lower them so that he can put one under each of her knees and help her to lift them upwards to change the angle that he's thrusting her from.

Tug of Love Sex Position

This position is one of a kind, and the last thing couples might actually dream of

The man first need to lie down on the bed on his back with his legs open. The woman then sits down on top of him and let him thrust into her vagina, with her legs on either side of him in front of her. Next She needs to start to lean backwards until she is lying down on the bed (she should put her arms behind her to ease herself down). Her head should be close to his feet. The woman can rest her legs on his chest or on either side of him, whichever is more comfortable.

Now that they are both lying down, the man should grab her hands so that he can pull her in towards him.

Victory Sex Position

The Victory is more or less the Missionary position but with the woman's legs extended out straight and forming into a v-shape toward the ceiling.

In this position, the woman simply lays down on her back while her partner lies face-down on top of her.

Viennese Oyster Sex Position

This sex position requires a great deal of flexibility. And most couples usually would get to a point where they can't continue due to the woman's inability to push past that point.

In this sex position the woman lays on her back with her lower back and legs raised all the way up so that her ankles are crossed behind her own head. The exact end position depends on the flexibility of the woman. This position totally exposes the groin of the woman to the man who lays on top the woman to penetrate. The man moves up and down on the woman to create friction. He needs to use his hands to support his own body weight so as not to crush his woman.

X Marks the Spot Sex Position

This sex position is really just a variation of the regular Missionary position. It's fun to try if the couple finds out that they are getting bored of Missionary and want something similar but more fun and different.

To perform it, the woman lays on her back while her man is on top. This position got its 'X' part from the fact that the bodies of the couples will form an X when viewed from above. So if the woman is lying down on her back with her feet at the end of the bed and her head at the top of the bed where the pillows usually are, her man will be lying across the bed, with his head by one side of the bed and his feet by the other side of the bed.

Bumper Cars Sex Position

This position is one very exotic position. To some couples this position is simple novel and to some others it is cool. Even the name is a little out of there.

The man must be sure to check that his penis is flexible enough. If he is standing up straight, then the man needs to be able to point his penis directly downwards towards the ground quite comfortably before even trying out this sex position.

If the man has enough flexibility, then you are good to go. Firstly the woman lies down on her stomach on the bed, with her legs straight and open wide. Then her man lies down on his stomach facing in completely the opposite direction and his legs straight and open wide as well. The man then reverses back towards the woman until his thighs are positioned over her thighs and he can pull his penis so that it's pointing towards her vagina. Then the man slowly needs penetrates the woman's vagina, making sure not to overstretch his penis.

Irish Garden Sex Position

The position is similar to the Betty Rocker position, very interesting and doesn't take a great deal of flexibility as it might look. It's very easy to perform.

The man sits down on the bed. He should have his back upright and straight, his legs out in front of him and also opened fairly wide. The man can bend his knees if he finds that more comfortable for him. The woman now gets down on all fours and reverses herself towards him. She will have to lower her waist down onto her man by straightening out her legs behind him (one on each side of his waist). Next she lowers her head and shoulders onto the bed until they are resting on it.

Jockey Sex Position

This position got its name from the idea that your man would like a horse riding jockey when in this position.

The woman lies with her face downwards on her bed with her legs together and straight. The man now straddles her with his knees on either side of her waist. The man then enters the woman either anally or vaginally and starts to thrust. He doesn't have to lean forward as a jockey would do when riding a race horse but he can if he wanted. He can also lean backwards slightly in the Jockey position. The man can also lean right on top of her so that it feels more like you are spooning with him.

Doggie Style

This position also known as rear entry is a great position that has enjoyed popularity over the years, maybe because it comes with this naughty feeling.

In this position, the man enters the woman's vagina from behind as she is on all fours on the bed or couch. This position supports very deep penetration, as the woman's body is already being so angled; so the g-spot can be stimulated by each penetration of the man's penis. Depending on how far bent over the woman is and how fast the man can thrust into his woman. His testicles will also slap against his woman's vagina which can be really very exciting. Stimulation of the Clitoris is also very possible by both the partners.

Superwoman Sex Position

This position may sound like one of those positions where the woman literally needs to do alot of work to be the 'Superwoman'. Luckily for her this is not the case at all, the man does most of the work. In some ways the Superwoman position is quite like the Life Raft position.

The woman lies down on your bed on her belly, with her arms resting on the bed, stretched out in front of her. While her stomach should be on the bed, her waist will be at the edge with her legs hanging over the side. The man will then penetrate the woman while standing from behind and will start thrusting in and out.

Basset Hound Sex Position

This position is a variation of the Doggy Style. It is named so because of the closeness of the couples to the floor. The position is straightforward; the woman is on all fours with the man holding on to the woman's bottom or the sides. Because of the low position the woman's rear is pushed right back, while the man's knees is placed to either